PARENTING

with Anxiety

Chapter 1: Introduction

Definition of Anxiety in Parenting: Anxiety is a mental health issue that affects people of all ages and socioeconomic backgrounds. Parents' worry can appear in a variety of ways, ranging from general concerns about their children's well-being to more specific anxieties about their own parental responsibilities. Understanding the spectrum of anxiety disorders is critical for understanding their impact in the context of parenting.

Types of Anxiety Disorders:

Anxiety disorders encompass a wide range of ailments, each with its own set of symptoms and triggers.

Generalized Anxiety Disorder (GAD) is defined by excessive and persistent anxiety over everyday matters such as future events, parenting decisions, and child safety.

Panic Disorder is characterized by acute and abrupt episodes of fear or panic, which are frequently accompanied by physical symptoms such as shortness of breath and a rapid heart rate. These incidents might disturb daily routines as well as parental responsibilities. certain phobias are irrational fears of certain items or events (such as driving, animals, or social situations) that can limit parental involvement in their children's activities or trips. Parents can effectively manage anxiety by recognizing their own symptoms and finding appropriate help and solutions based on an awareness of these diseases.

Social Anxiety Disorder is characterized by an extreme fear of social circumstances and criticism from others, which influences parental interactions in social settings such as playgrounds or school functions.

This section looks at how anxiety affects several aspects of parenting.

Parenting methods: Anxiety can influence parenting methods by making people more cautious or protective of decisions. The problems that parents face in balancing safety and independence may have an impact on their children's growth and autonomy.

Decision-Making Processes: Self-doubt and reluctance caused by anxiety are common characteristics of the decision-making process. Anxiety can interfere with daily relationships with children by reducing communication, emotional reactivity, consistency in support and direction, and the capacity to make simple decisions such as selecting extracurricular activities or addressing disciplinary concerns. These judgments may also have an impact on children's experiences and result in delays in action.

Typical Obstacles Faced by Anxious Parents:

Stress Management: Exacerbating typical stressors can make it challenging for parents to maintain emotional balance and resilience in their parenting tasks.

Consistency Preservation: Anxiety-induced uncertainties and anxieties can decrease consistency in parental activities, such as rule and boundary setting.

Family Dynamics: Anxiety can affect spousal relationships and sibling connections. Understanding these challenges allows parents to actively explore solutions and support systems that promote resilience and good parenting practices despite their worry.

Chapter 2: Understanding Anxiety Disorders: A Comprehensive Overview

Anxiety disorders are a group of diseases that can have a significant influence on daily life and parenthood. When anxiety-related stressors are prevalent, parents may struggle to provide a harmonious and supportive atmosphere. Understanding these diseases is critical for parents so that they may detect their own symptoms, seek appropriate care, and implement effective coping techniques.

For example, generalized anxiety disorder (GAD) is distinguished by excessive and persistent worry about a variety of life tasks, including parental responsibilities. Parents with Generalized Anxiety Disorder (GAD) may struggle to manage day-to-day tasks and experience increased stress as a result of their continual fear of potential threats or negative consequences for their children.

Panic Disorder is characterized by frequent, unexpected panic attacks that are followed by intense worry or discomfort.

The characteristic of social anxiety disorder (SAD) is intense fear of social situations and scrutiny from others. These episodes can be extremely draining, affecting parental responsibilities and interactions with children under stressful situations. These events might occur suddenly.

Specific phobias are defined by unreasonable dread of particular things or circumstances. Parents with SAD may avoid attending social activities or engaging in parent-child interactions in public places, limiting their ability to actively participate in their children's social development.

For parents, this may encompass apprehensions regarding particular parenting activities or environments, such as the dread of driving with children or the fear of animals that may impede family outings and activities. Parents are able to identify their own symptoms and triggers by comprehending these anxiety disorders, which in turn enables them to develop effective management strategies and early intervention.

 Anxiety is characterized by a range of physical and psychological symptoms that can fluctuate in intensity and frequency:

Symptoms of the Body: A common physical manifestation of anxiety is a rapid heartbeat, which can exacerbate feelings of tension and discomfort.

Perspiration: Anxiety frequently induces excessive perspiration, which can be observed in stressful parenting situations. Anxiety can result in muscle tension, which can result in physical exhaustion and discomfort.

Symptoms of a psychological nature: Uncontrollable and persistent anxiety regarding future outcomes, child safety, and parenting decisions is referred to as excessive concern.

Irritability: Parent-child interactions may be adversely affected by increased anxiety, which can result in irritability and impatience.

Concentration difficulties: Anxiety can impede focus and concentration, which can make it difficult to complete daily tasks efficiently.

Anxiety Triggers: It is imperative for parents to comprehend the triggers that exacerbate anxiety symptoms in order to proactively manage their condition.

Parenting Stressors: Anxiety symptoms can be induced by everyday parenting responsibilities, including the management of schedules, the discipline of children, and the balance between work and family life.

Conflicts Within the Family: Stress and anxiety levels may be elevated by disagreements or conflicts with co-parents or extended family members.

External Pressures: Anxiety may be exacerbated by financial concerns, societal expectations, and pressures associated with children's academic or social accomplishments.

Parents can effectively manage anxiety by developing personalized strategies and seeking professional support by recognizing these symptoms and triggers. This understanding serves as the foundation for building a loving environment for caregivers and children, as well as implementing coping techniques.

Chapter 3: The Difficulties of Anxiety-Related Parenting and Their Impact on Parenting Style

Anxiety-related parenting presents unique obstacles that can have a substantial impact on parenting strategies and approaches. This chapter investigates how anxiety influences parents' decision-making and behaviors, which in turn affects a variety of aspects of childrearing:

Difficulties with Risk Acceptance: Anxious parents frequently find it difficult to allow their children to participate in age-appropriate activities and risks. Fear of potential injury or mishaps can lead to overprotective behavior, limiting children's opportunity for independent learning and discovery.

Difficulty Establishing Boundaries: Anxiety-related stress can make it difficult for parents to constantly establish clear norms and boundaries.

Discipline Enforcement Obstacles: Anxiety can make it difficult to regularly enforce discipline. This can influence children's behavior and comprehension of expectations. Anxiety-induced hesitations or uncertainties regarding appropriate penalties might lead to uneven disciplinary actions. Understanding these dynamics enables parents to identify how anxiety influences their parenting style and relationships with their children.

It can be difficult for parents to remain cool and forceful during disciplinary interactions, which might result in poor disciplinary techniques or garbled messages.

Concerns About Anxiety Transmission to Children:

Parents frequently express concern about the prospect of their children inheriting anxiety, taking into consideration both environmental and genetic variables.

Hereditary Predisposition: According to research, anxiety disorders may have a hereditary component, increasing the risk of similar illnesses developing in offspring if one or both parents are anxious.

Parents can lessen the impact of anxiety on their parenting practices by identifying specific issues and implementing measures. Understanding this innate risk factor promotes proactive measures to improve children's mental health and emotional resilience.

Environmental Factors: Family dynamics, parenting methods, and stress exposure are some of the environmental factors that might influence children's anxiety. The emotional development and stress management capabilities of children are substantially determined by the anxiety levels and coping mechanisms of their parents.

Strategies to Reduce the Impact on Children:

Parents may employ the following strategies to mitigate the emotional impact of their anxiety on their children:

Fostering Open Communication: By establishing a supportive environment in which children are encouraged to express their emotions and concerns, emotional awareness and resilience are cultivated.

Modeling Healthy Coping Behaviors: Children acquire adaptive coping skills by observing effective stress management techniques, including deep breathing, mindfulness, and problem-solving.

Seeking Professional Assistance: Consulting with mental health professionals can offer advice on parental strategies and interventions that can be used to promote the emotional well-being of children.

Parents can significantly contribute to the improvement of their children's emotional resilience and the reduction of the potential negative effects of anxiety on their development by addressing these concerns and employing proactive strategies.

Chapter 4: Anxiety Management Strategies

Effective strategies are required to manage symptoms and foster emotional well-being when parenting with anxiety. This chapter delves into professional interventions and practical methods for helping parents manage their anxiety and improve their parenting experience.

The first step in managing anxiety is to prioritize self-care and adopt healthy coping mechanisms that are tailored to each individual's unique needs.

1. Regular exercise releases neurotransmitters that can reduce anxiety symptoms and improve overall well-being;

2. Adequate Sleep: Maintaining a regular sleep schedule and practicing good sleep hygiene can improve overall well-being and stress resilience;

3. Mindfulness Practices: Techniques such as yoga, meditation, and deep breathing exercises can help reduce anxiety and promote relaxation.

4. Relaxation methods, such as progressive muscle relaxation and guided visualization, are useful for relieving physical stress and encouraging relaxation.

Implementing these personal coping methods allows parents to proactively control anxiety symptoms and increase their capacity to engage positively with their children.

Cognitive-Behavioral Techniques (CBT): Cognitive restructuring is the process of identifying and confronting negative thought patterns that contribute to anxiety, and then replacing them with more realistic and balanced perspectives.

Seeking Professional Assistance: Recognizing the importance of professional counsel and intervention is critical for properly managing anxiety.

Cognitive-Behavioral Therapy (CBT): This rigorous therapeutic approach assists clients in identifying and changing detrimental thought patterns and behaviors that cause anxiety. It provides parents with the necessary skills to manage stress and improve their coping strategies.

The second step is called exposure therapy, a treatment method in which people are gradually exposed to anxiety-provoking experiences in a safe and controlled environment. It enables parents to confront and conquer certain phobias and anxieties related to their job as parents.

Step Three consists of acceptance and commitment therapy, or ACT, aims to help people commit to activities that are consistent with their beliefs, while also emphasizing the importance of mindfulness and tolerating problematic thoughts and feelings.

Parents can reduce anxiety by assisting their children in developing psychological flexibility and resilience.

Things to Consider When Managing Medication: Doctors may give medication to alleviate severe anxiety symptoms.

To examine the potential benefits and drawbacks of pharmaceutical treatment, as well as prescription options, consult with a healthcare practitioner, such as a primary care physician or psychiatrist.

Chapter 5: Techniques and Advice for Parents

Intentional techniques are required to create a supporting network, maintain consistency, and foster positive interactions with children when parenting with anxiety. Parents can effectively manage anxiety, increase resilience, and create a supportive environment conducive to positive parental experiences by combining personal coping techniques and seeking professional help.

If anxiety significantly inhibits everyday functioning, interferes with parental responsibilities, or creates distressing symptoms that reduce quality of life, parents should seek professional help.

This chapter delves into the practical strategies and suggestions that can be utilized to improve parenting effectiveness while also managing anxiety:

Open Communication with Children: Good communication creates the framework for recognizing and reducing anxiety in the family dynamic.

Maintaining Environmental Safety: Creating a judgment-free, transparent environment in which children can freely express their anxiety-related feelings and concerns. Encourage regular conversations about emotions and give children the opportunity to ask and receive responses.

Age-appropriate communication regarding anxiety should be tailored to children's developmental stages and cognitive abilities. Use age-appropriate words and examples to help the youngster realize that worry is a common emotion that everyone experiences.

Establishing Boundaries and Routines: Consistency and structure provide stability and reduce anxiety triggers for both parents and children. Children can be effectively enabled to control their own anxiety by emphasizing resilience and problem-solving abilities.

Developing Trust: Children can build resilience in the face of anxiety-related issues by developing trust, improving parent-child relationships, and promoting emotional intelligence through open communication. Parents can reassure children by sharing their own anxiety experiences and modeling healthy coping skills.

Maintaining Consistent Parenting Practices: Regular mealtimes, bedtimes, and assignment schedules make youngsters feel safe and stable. Similarly, implementing regular norms and punishments helps children grasp what is expected of them and reduces the anxiety associated with uncertainty.

Creating Realistic Expectations: When creating objectives and expectations for children, it is vital to consider their unique strengths and shortcomings. By adjusting expectations to match children's developmental stages and skills, a supportive environment that supports growth and performance is created.

Structure Flexibility: By allowing for flexibility within established routines, parents can respond to changing situations while maintaining overall structure and consistency. Parental involvement in decision-making processes and communication of changes fosters a sense of empowerment and autonomy in children. The establishment of protocols and boundaries promotes a loving environment, which improves family unity and children's mental health.

Establishing a Support Network: To effectively manage anxiety and preserve general well-being, parents must first establish a support network.

Seeking Family Support: Promoting open discussion about anxiety-related issues and parenting challenges with partners, extended family, and close friends. Sharing duties and asking for help when needed encourages collaborative problem-solving and strengthens familial bonds.

Support Groups and Community options: Investigate local options such as parenting classes, counseling services, and support groups for anxious parents. Joining online forums and support groups allows parents to connect with other parents facing similar challenges, share experiences, and offer support to one another.

Establishing a strong support network enables parents to overcome barriers, minimize feelings of isolation, and have access to tools that promote emotional resilience and general well-being.

Chapter 6: Building a Healthy Environment

The process of parenting with anxiety entails building a loving atmosphere that promotes emotional resilience and well-being in both parents and children. To effectively treat anxiety-related concerns, consider consulting with mental health professionals such as therapists or counselors for individual or family therapy sessions.

Looking for guidance from healthcare specialists to seek specialized support and strategies geared specifically to manage parental anxiety. The primary goals of this chapter are to illustrate healthy coping skills, promote resilience, and maintain a supportive family dynamic.

Parents' actions and responses have a major impact on their children's anxiety-related attitudes and behaviors. Healthy coping methods, such as deep breathing exercises, mindfulness exercises, and positive self-talk, have been shown to effectively manage stress and anxiety. Active participation in stress-relieving activities such as hobbies, physical exercise, or creative outlets reinforces the significance of self-care and emotional regulation.

Emotional Openness: Encouraging open discussions about anxiety-related events and emotions helps to normalize these experiences within the family. Sharing personal difficulties with anxiety at an appropriate age can assist family members build empathy, understanding, and mutual support.

Resilience and Vulnerability in Balance: Parents help their children develop effective anxiety-management skills and resilience throughout their lives by encouraging emotional awareness and modeling appropriate coping habits. Children learn to address issues in a proactive and composed manner by displaying adaptive problem-solving abilities.

The cultivation of critical thinking and resilience in the handling of anxiety-provoking situations is aided by encouraging ideation and the investigation of numerous solutions in partnership. Openness about parental barriers demonstrates authenticity and vulnerability by expressing personal experiences with anxiety in a constructive and age-appropriate manner. This fosters a supportive family atmosphere by emphasizing that anxiety is a normal emotion and discussing coping techniques and support systems.

Encouraging children to communicate their emotions and fears helps them develop emotional intelligence and self-awareness. Reassuring and validating children's emotions also promotes resilience and confidence in their abilities to manage anxiety-related situations.

Building Stronger Families: **By sharing experiences and encouraging one another, families can become more supportive and cohesive. Participating in family activities that foster empathy, cooperation, and constructive communication enhances family bonds and resilience.**

By establishing a balance between vulnerability and resilience, parents provide a safe environment in which children feel comfortable exploring their emotions, learning coping methods, and confronting obstacles head on.

Chapter 7: Addressing Challenges at Different Parenting Stages

This chapter examines the particular issues of parenting anxious children. This chapter delves into the ways that can be utilized to successfully address these challenges at various phases of parenting.

Early Childhood: Attachment and emotional development are especially important in a child's early years. Parents usually encounter the following challenges:

Separation anxiety and the promotion of emotional stability. Separation anxiety management is validating and accepting the anxiety that children experience when they transition to a new daycare, preschool, or other setting. Providing reassurance that they will be safe and return, as well as establishing predictable routines, can help children feel less worried and more emotionally secure.

Improving Emotional Well-Being: Emotional attachments are formed by supporting positive parent-child interactions through storytelling, play, and loving activities. Providing a loving and caring environment in which children feel appreciated and respected boosts their self-esteem and emotional strength.

Parental Coping Mechanisms: Applying self-care techniques, such as mindfulness exercises and seeking out social support, to reduce the stress and anxiety that are frequently linked to early childhood parenting; consulting pediatricians or early childhood educators for guidance on age-appropriate techniques and interventions; In the early years, parents lay the groundwork for their child's healthy emotional development by addressing separation anxiety and fostering emotions. Parents who are dealing with anxiety must offer their teenagers with the support they require while still encouraging autonomy.

Encouraging Self-Sufficiency: Allowing teenagers to make age-appropriate decisions and accept responsibility for their actions increases autonomy and self-esteem. Finding the right amount of independence, support, and encouragement helps teenagers develop resilience and confidence.

Open Communication About Mental Health: Normalizing discussions about stress, academic pressures, and social challenges promotes a supportive family atmosphere while reducing stigma. Teenagers are encouraged to express their emotions and seek help if needed. This includes initiating open discussions about mental health, especially anxiety.

Promoting healthy lifestyle choices such as frequent physical activity, appropriate sleep, and balanced nutrition can help with stress management and general well-being. To help their adolescents develop resilience and adaptive coping skills, parents must strike a balance between support and independence while navigating adolescence with anxiety.

Parents can establish a caring environment that promotes emotional well-being and builds parent-child connections by addressing the unique problems of early childhood and adolescence with intentional tactics and support. In this book, we've looked at a variety of ways and approaches for managing anxiety, fostering great relationships, and promoting emotional wellness.

Chapter 8: Conclusion

This final chapter provides a summary of the most significant insights and concludes with final reflections on the challenges of parenting while dealing with anxiety:

Challenges and Strategies Summary

Anxiety and Parenting: Anxiety disorders are classified into four categories: generalized anxiety disorder, panic disorder, social anxiety disorder, and specific phobias.

Influence on parents: Effects on daily interactions with children, decision-making processes, and parental styles.Concerns Regarding the Transmission of Anxiety: The emotional development of children is influenced by both genetic predispositions and environmental factors.

Strategies for Effectively Managing Anxiety: **Personal Coping Mechanisms:** Cognitive-behavioral techniques (CBT), mindfulness practices, and self-care routines.

Seeking Professional Assistance: **Medication management, exposure therapy, and cognitive-behavioral therapy (CBT) under the supervision of a professional.**

Tips and Strategies for Parenting: **Establishing routines and boundaries, fostering open communication, and establishing a support network.**

CONCLUDING THOUGHTS

A journey that necessitates ongoing self-awareness, resilience, and adaptation is that of parenting with anxiety. Parenting with anxiety is a challenging process that needs proactive management of anxiety symptoms, as well as self-compassion and patience. To provide a loving atmosphere for their children, parents must first prioritize their own mental health and well-being.

Ongoing Assistance: **Parents are encouraged to seek help from mental health experts, community services, and loved ones.**

Resilience-Building: **Emphasizing the significance of problem-solving skills, encouraging open conversation about emotions, and demonstrating appropriate coping strategies.**

Remembering that parenting tactics may need to alter as children grow and develop necessitates adapting parenting approaches to meet their evolving requirements. Prioritizing mental health and using the practices outlined in this book can help parents establish a loving atmosphere in which both themselves and their children can thrive emotionally and interpersonally. As you continue your parenting experience, remember that resilience and asking for help are vital strategies for facing the difficulties of parenthood with anxiety.

Accept each day with courage and compassion, knowing that you are contributing to your family's happiness and well-being. I wish your trip is full with enjoyable, enlightening, and developing experiences.